MACROBIOTIC

DIET

FOR NOVICES

Enriched Recipes, Foods, Meal Plan & Procedures That Focuses On Body Nourishment, Stress Reduction, Approach To Macrobiotic Wellness And More

DR. MATEO GABRIEL

DISCLAIMER

The information in this book is only meant to be used for general reading. In any way, the author and publisher do not promise or represent that the information in this work is full, correct, reliable, appropriate, or available. This includes any warranties that are expressed or implied. Because of this, you should only rely on this material at your own risk.

This book is not meant to replace professional help. If you have any questions about a subject, you should always get help from a qualified expert. The author and distributor of this book are not responsible for how the information in it is used or abused.

The author's thoughts and feelings are shown in this book. They do not necessarily represent the official policy or stance of any other person, group, employer, or business.

Any third-party material that you can get to through this book is not endorsed or backed by the author or publisher.

The information in this book is correct at the time it was published, after all possible checks. However, the author and distributor are not responsible for any loss, damage, or inconvenience that may be caused by mistakes or omissions.

TABLE OF CONTENTS

CHAPTER ONE

INTRODUCTION TO MACROBIOTIC DIET

COMPREHENDING ROBOTICS

Macrobotics, which embodies the combination of mechanical engineering, computer science, and artificial intelligence, is a cutting-edge field at the convergence of robotics and macro-scale applications. The goal of this emerging field is to investigate and create robotic systems that do activities that require significant physical dimensions or environmental problems, sometimes on a greater scale than traditional robots. It is possible to break down the phrase

"Macrobotics" to determine its fundamental meaning: "macro" refers to large-scale, and "robotics" is the field of study that deals with the creation, maintenance, use, and application of robots.

MEANING AND HISTORY

The roots of Macrobotics can be found in the changing needs of industry and other fields that require large-scale automation. The need for robots that could handle heavier weights and navigate challenging surroundings emerged as industries looked to increase productivity, save costs, and tackle jobs that presented serious difficulties for human labor. This led to the progression of micro-scale robotics into the creation of systems that could manage macro-scale tasks, which is how macrobiotics got their start.

FUNDAMENTALS AND PHILOSOPHIES

The fundamental ideas of robotics, artificial intelligence, and mechanical engineering form the basis of macrobiotics. These concepts include the development of strong mechanical structures that can support heavy loads, the incorporation of complex sensor systems for the observation of the surrounding environment, and the application of cutting-edge algorithms for autonomous operation and decision-making. Unlike their smaller counterparts, macrobots frequently encounter particular difficulties with dynamics, stability, and power consumption, calling for creative solutions that defy accepted paradigms in robotics design.

From a philosophical standpoint, macrobiotics welcome the notion of using technology to augment human labor and do jobs that traditional automation cannot handle. The ideology includes the idea that we can build systems that work in concert with machines and people to tackle difficult problems. These problems can range from large-scale industrial operations to disaster response and extreme environment research. Ensuring the proper use of these technologies, preventing potential misuse, and addressing concerns about job displacement and societal effects are the ethical aspects underlying Macrobiotics.

Macrobotics represents a frontier in technological development, stretching the limits of what large-scale robots are capable of. Its definition, which combines the terms "macro" and "robotics," demonstrates a dedication to tackling problems that call for a more substantial physical presence. Macrobotics' interdisciplinary nature is emphasized by its principles and philosophy, which link the field's roots to the changing demands of various industries. The field's goal is to advance large-scale robotic systems through innovation, responsibility, and collaboration.

CHAPTER TWO

ADVANTAGES OF AUTOMATED FOOD PROCESSING

BETTER HEALTH

Consuming plant-based and minimally processed foods is known as macrobiotic eating, and it has been demonstrated to have significant positive effects on general health. This meal plan has a strong emphasis on a wide variety of whole grains, legumes, fruits, and vegetables since they are high in fiber, antioxidants, and other nutrients. Together, these components support better digestion, stronger immunity, and a lower chance of developing chronic illnesses like diabetes, heart disease, and some types of cancer.

The ability of macrobiotic consumption to control blood sugar levels is one of its main benefits. Whole meals include complex carbs that release glucose gradually, avoiding abrupt blood sugar rises and crashes. This consistency aids in maintaining energy levels throughout the day and can be especially helpful for people with diabetes or those trying to avoid developing the disease.

Moreover, the macrobiotic eating pattern's emphasis on plant-based proteins offers a healthy substitute for animal proteins, which may reduce the risk of cardiovascular problems. Plant-based diets may help lower blood pressure and cholesterol, and enhance heart health, according to research.

ECO-FRIENDLY LIFESTYLE

Macrobiotic eating is an environmentally beneficial substitute for typical diets, and it is consistent with the ideas of sustainable living. Compared to the production of animal-based products, the production of plant-based foods often requires fewer natural resources, such as land and water. Macrobiotic eating habits are one way that people help to lessen their ecological impact.

A typical component of macrobiotic eating is the habit of sourcing locally and seasonally, which further reduces the environmental effect of long-distance food transportation. This regional strategy helps regional farmers and promotes the expansion of sustainable farming methods.

A macrobiotic diet's decreased reliance on highly processed foods also lessens the environmental impact of the manufacture, packaging, and shipping of these goods. Selecting whole, plant-based diets is frequently a more environmentally responsible and sustainable method of providing nutrition for the body.

MAINTAINING WEIGHT

Macrobiotic eating offers a comprehensive and well-rounded strategy for people looking for efficient weight-management techniques. The focus on nutrient-dense, whole meals guarantees a broad spectrum of vital vitamins and minerals and aids in calorie management. When properly designed, plant-based diets are generally lower in calories and saturated fats, which makes them beneficial for both weight loss and maintenance.

The high fiber content of macrobiotic diets is essential for encouraging fullness, lowering total caloric intake, and maintaining intestinal health. In addition to avoiding overly processed and sugary foods, this helps to make weight control more stable and long-lasting.

Furthermore, a macrobiotic diet's wide range of nutrients promotes metabolic processes and gives the body the resources it needs for effective energy use. This can promote a positive and long-lasting attitude to general well-being by resulting in weight loss as well as the long-term maintenance of a healthy weight.

CHAPTER THREE

THE MACROBIOTIC DIET'S BASIS

BOTH MICRO AND MACRONUTRIENTS

One of the cornerstones of the Foundations of Macrobiotic Diet understands macro and micronutrients, which are essential for maintaining general health and well-being. The body needs both macro and micronutrients in different amounts to function properly. These nutrients ensure the body's energy production, growth, and maintenance by acting as the building blocks for physiological activities.

As the name implies, macronutrients are nutrients that are needed in greater amounts. They consist of lipids, proteins, and carbs. The body uses carbohydrates as its main energy source to power numerous internal processes. Proteins are essential for hormone and enzyme synthesis, muscle growth, and tissue repair. Contrary to popular belief, fats are necessary for the synthesis of hormones, proper brain function, and the absorption of fat-soluble vitamins.

KNOWLEDGE OF MACRONUTRIENTS

Recognizing the importance of preserving a proper ratio between carbs, proteins, and fats is a necessary part of understanding macronutrients. Maintaining this equilibrium is crucial for enhancing metabolic functions and guaranteeing that the organism gets a sufficient and diverse range of nutrients. The exact nutritional needs of an individual can change depending on their age, sex, degree of exercise, and general health.

Micronutrients are an essential component of the macrobiotic diet, along with macronutrients. Micronutrients include vitamins and minerals, which are required in lesser amounts but are just as important for preserving good health.

Essential ideas like the Energy Balance Equation, Caloric Intake, and Expenditure, and Finding the Right Balance for Your Goals are at the center of The Foundations of Macrobiotic Diet. It is essential to comprehend these ideas to create a diet plan that works and supports personal fitness and health goals.

THE EQUATION FOR ENERGY BALANCE

The Macrobiotic Diet philosophy is based on the Energy Balance Equation. The link between the energy obtained from food and the energy used for physical activity and metabolic processes is highlighted by this basic idea. A balance between calories burnt and calories consumed is crucial for achieving optimal health and weight management. A calorie surplus causes weight gain, whereas a calorie shortage causes weight loss.

CONSUMPTION AND INTAKE OF CALORIES

Important roles are played by calorie intake and expenditure in the energy balance equation. Caloric intake is the quantity of calories consumed from food and drink, whereas caloric expenditure includes the energy used by physical activity, basal metabolic rate, and the thermic effect of food. Finding the ideal balance between these two elements is essential for reaching particular fitness and health objectives, such as muscular growth, weight reduction, or maintenance.

CHOOSING THE CORRECT BALANCE FOR YOUR OBJECTIVES

A customized strategy for calorie intake and expenditure is required to Find the Right Balance for Your Goals. Since every person has different activity levels, metabolic rates, and fitness goals, it is crucial to customize the Macrobiotic Diet to meet each person's demands. Age, gender, body composition, and the quantity and frequency of physical exercise all play a role in finding the ideal balance. To achieve the desired results and optimize energy balance, it is important to customize the intake of total calories and macronutrient ratios.

The Foundations of Macrobiotic Diet concludes by highlighting the importance of Finding the Right Balance for Your Goals, Caloric Intake and Expenditure, and the Energy Balance Equation. A comprehensive comprehension of these ideas enables people to make knowledgeable food decisions, opening the door to long-term improvements in fitness and health.

NUTRITION BASED ON PLANTS

A key tenet of the Macrobiotic Diet is Plant-Based Nutrition, which emphasizes consuming a range of foods originating from plants to meet nutritional demands. This method focuses on using fruits, vegetables, grains, legumes, nuts, and seeds as the main food sources. These plant-based diets support general health and well-being because they are high in vital elements like vitamins, minerals, fiber, and antioxidants.

THE VALUE OF PLANT-BASED DIETS

It is impossible to exaggerate the significance of including plant-based foods in the Macrobiotic Diet. Many health advantages of a plant-based diet have been linked to it, including a lower chance of developing chronic illnesses including diabetes, heart disease, and some types of cancer. The body's natural defense mechanisms and the promotion of proper physiological function are greatly aided by the plethora of phytochemicals and bioactive substances present in plants.

The Macrobiotic Diet's focus on plant-based nourishment is consistent with the idea of creating a sustainable and well-balanced eating routine. In addition to being high in nutrients, plants are also less harmful to the environment and use fewer resources than diets based on animals. A wide range of nutrients is ensured by including a variety of plant-based foods in the diet, which supports general health and vigor.

MAJOR SOURCES OF NUTRIENTS

A range of plant-based foods are important sources of nutrients in the Macrobiotic Diet and are great suppliers of key vitamins and minerals. Rich in calcium and iron, leafy greens like spinach and kale support healthy bones and blood oxygen delivery. Complex carbs, fiber, and B vitamins are included in whole grains like brown rice and quinoa, which support prolonged energy release and nervous system function.

Legumes, which include beans and lentils, are a key part of the Macrobiotic Diet since they are excellent providers of vitamins, fiber, and protein. Nuts and seeds, including flaxseeds, chia seeds, and almonds, provide protein, healthy fats, and omega-3 fatty acids that support brain and cardiovascular health.

Plant-Based Nutrition is emphasized in the Foundations of Macrobiotic Diet as the cornerstone for general health. Designing a sustainable and well-balanced meal that adheres to the Macrobiotic meal's tenets requires an understanding of the significance of plant-based foods and the identification of important nutritional sources.

CHAPTER FOUR

FUNDAMENTALS OF MACROBOTIC CONSUMPTION

THE PLATE MACROBOTIC

A key idea in the field of the macrobiotic diet is the Macrobiotic Plate, which emphasizes a comprehensive and well-balanced approach to nutrition. In contrast to conventional dietary patterns that could emphasize certain nutrients or rigorous calorie tracking, the Macrobiotic Plate invites people to think about the whole makeup of their meals. Usually, the plate is split into pieces that correspond to various dietary groups, with a focus on striking a balance between fats, proteins, and carbohydrates.

MAINTAINING A BALANCE AMONG CARBS, PROTEINS, AND FATS

The foundation of macrobiotic eating ideas is the balance of fats, proteins, and carbohydrates. The body uses fats for many biological processes, proteins for muscle growth and repair, and carbohydrates for energy. To guarantee a varied and nutrient-rich diet, the Macrobiotic Plate emphasizes the significance of incorporating whole, unprocessed foods in each category. Whole grains, such as quinoa and brown rice, frequently serve as the basis for the section on carbohydrates, with beans, legumes, and plant-based proteins serving as the part's protein source. To round off the balanced plate, healthy fats are added from places like nuts and avocados.

RATIOS ADJUSTED FOR INDIVIDUAL NEEDS

Reducing ratios to suit individual needs recognizes that people have different nutritional demands depending on their age, degree of exercise, and health. The Macrobiotic Plate's adaptability enables customization to satisfy these unique requirements. While some people may benefit from a little higher protein intake for muscle maintenance, others may need a higher amount of carbohydrates for sustained energy. Because of its versatility, the Macrobiotic Plate is a flexible and inclusive approach to nutrition that can be customized to fit a range of lifestyles and health objectives.

The Macrobiotic Plate also supports the idea of mindful eating, which encourages people to pay attention to their bodies' signals and react to signs of hunger and fullness. In addition to encouraging physical well-being, this holistic approach fosters a closer relationship with both the environment and one's own body. The Macrobiotic Plate promotes general health and wellness by emphasizing food quality and nutrient balance. It provides a practical and sustainable way to make dietary decisions.

The Macrobiotic Plate offers a thorough foundation for a balanced diet by emphasizing the balancing of carbohydrates, proteins, and fats while allowing for individuality. This method encourages a conscious and flexible approach to bodily nourishment that can be customized to meet individual requirements and tastes, going beyond simple calorie monitoring. The Macrobiotic Plate integrates entire, nutrient-dense meals to provide a practical guide for people looking for a sustainable and comprehensive approach to nutrition.

CONSCIOUS EATING

A key idea in the macrobiotic eating theory is mindful eating, which emphasizes a purposeful and mindful attitude to food consumption. It entails increasing awareness of one's thoughts and emotions surrounding eating, paying attention to the sensory components of food, and being present during the eating experience. A holistic approach to well-being is fostered by macrobiotic eating, which places equal emphasis on the entire eating experience as well as the food's nutritional value.

THE RELATIONSHIP BETWEEN NUTRITION AND MINDFULNESS

One essential component of macrobiotic eating practices is the relationship between nutrition and awareness. By encouraging people to eat with complete awareness, mindfulness helps people get a better knowledge of their nutritional needs and how their food choices affect their general health. Eating in the present moment might help people become more conscious of their bodies' reactions to various nutrients and feel more grateful for the nourishment that food provides.

USEFUL ADVICE FOR MINDFUL EATING

An integral part of the macrobiotic eating philosophy is a set of doable recommendations for mindful eating. These suggestions function as guides to assist people in integrating mindfulness into their regular eating practices. Turning off electronics and concentrating only on the process of eating is one sensible way to eat without interruptions. A deeper connection with the flavors and textures of food is made possible by chewing food properly and appreciating each bite, which makes eating more fulfilling and nourishing.

COMBINING FOODS FOR THE BEST DIGESTION

According to Principles of Macrobiotic Eating, food pairing is crucial for optimum digestion. This strategy is consistent with the notion that some meals enhance one another's flavor profiles, facilitate digestion, and enhance general health. The idea behind food combining is that various foods require different digestion environments, and by deliberately combining foods, you can improve the efficiency of your digestive system.

The Principles of Macrobiotic Eating place a strong emphasis on mixing foods in a way that facilitates the best possible digestion. For instance, it's often advised to combine proteins with non-starchy vegetables because their digestive needs differ. While non-starchy veggies digest more readily in an alkaline environment, proteins frequently require an acidic environment. Combining these two kinds of meals might help the digestive system work more effectively, which may lessen the chance of experiencing discomfort in the digestive tract.

INCREASING UPTAKE OF NUTRIENTS

The emphasis on improving nutrient absorption through thoughtful food pairings is another essential idea. Some nutrients are absorbed more easily when eaten with particular dietary groups. To improve the absorption of iron, for example, combine foods high in vitamin C, like citrus fruits or bell peppers, with foods high in iron, like leafy greens or legumes. By strategically combining these, the body can absorb nutrients to the fullest, promoting general health and energy.

TYPICAL FOOD MIXTURES

Another recommendation made by the Principles of Macrobiotic Eating is to be aware of typical food pairings that facilitate the body's natural digestion processes. For example, it's usually advised to avoid fermentation and digestive problems by eating fruits as a snack or on an empty stomach. Conversely, eating carbs with veggies or proteins can help control blood sugar levels and provide you with energy for the entire day. These recommendations are meant to maximize nutrient utilization and are based on an understanding of the body's digestion cycle.

The Principles of Macrobiotic Eating conclude by stressing the need for food combinations for the best possible digestion and absorption of nutrients.

CHAPTER FIVE
ORGANIZING MACROBIOTIC DINNERS

MEAL PLANNING TECHNIQUES

For macrobiotic meal prep to be smooth and effective, careful planning and calculated measures must be taken. Preparation and batch cooking are important tactics. Using this strategy, a large amount of food is prepared all at once, usually on one day of the week, to make a stockpile of readily assembled or ready-to-eat meals for the coming days. Not only can batch cooking saves you time every week, but it also guarantees that you'll always have access to well-balanced, healthful macrobiotic choices without having to cook every day.

PREPARING AHEAD AND COOKING IN BATCHES

You may optimize your time in the kitchen by including batch cooking into your meal planning regimen. This method entails choosing a range of macrobiotic components and preparing them in large quantities. For instance, you may prepare a protein source like beans or tofu, roast a variety of vegetables, and cook a big batch of quinoa. After cooking, these ingredients can be kept apart and rearranged in various ways to make a variety of tasty macrobiotic dinners throughout the week.

Another essential component of macrobiotic meal prep success is planning. This entails planning your weekly meals taking your taste preferences, nutritional requirements, and timetable into account. Achieving a balance between macronutrients while planning is crucial to guaranteeing sufficient consumption of healthy fats, proteins, and carbohydrates. Including a range of whole grains, legumes, veggies, and plant-based meats in your meals will help you achieve this.

FORMULATING EQUILIBRIUM WEEKLY MENUS

For macrobiotic meals to help you achieve and maintain maximum health, a weekly menu that is well-balanced is essential. It's crucial to include a variety of nutrient-dense meals from several food categories in a balanced menu. For instance, you may organize meals that include a range of bright vegetables, plant-based proteins like lentils or chickpeas, and healthful grains like brown rice or quinoa. This guarantees a fulfilling and joyful eating experience in addition to offering a range of vital nutrients.

In addition, a varied weekly menu guarantees that you get a wide variety of vitamins, minerals, and antioxidants while also preventing boredom. To add diversity to your macrobiotic dinners, think about integrating seasonal veggies, experimenting with different cooking techniques, and changing your protein sources. This method not only improves the nutritional value of your meals but also stimulates your palate and encourages sustained macrobiotic lifestyle adhesion.

Preparation for macrobiotic meals requires a combination of quantity cooking, planning ahead, and designing weekly menus that are well-balanced. These techniques help create a sustained and pleasurable macrobiotic eating experience in addition to saving time. You may promote a healthy and fulfilling macrobiotic lifestyle by thoughtfully organizing your meals and including a wide variety of nutrient-dense foods.

MACROFOBIC COOKBOOKS

The idea of macrobiotic meals is to develop nutrient-dense dishes that are customized to match particular macronutrient requirements. This entails carefully balancing the body's needs for lipids, proteins, and carbs to provide the best possible nourishment. Whole, unprocessed foods are frequently the main emphasis of macrobiotic recipes, which include a range of items to provide a complete nutritional profile. The macrobiotic meal planning ideas are in line with the emphasis on accuracy and efficiency.

BREAKFAST CONCEPTS

Macrorobotic meals are designed to jump-start the metabolism and give continuous energy throughout the morning. The macro bowl is a well-liked option that combines lean proteins like tofu or quinoa, healthy fats like avocado or nuts, and complex carbohydrates like quinoa or sweet potatoes. This provides the body with nourishment and establishes a healthy foundation for the rest of the day. Another go-to option is smoothie bowls, which combine a variety of fruits, veggies, and protein sources and provide a quick and easy approach to achieving macronutrient objectives while satisfying individual taste preferences.

OPTIONS FOR LUNCH AND DINNER

The nutrient-dense components used in macrobiotic lunches and dinners are carefully chosen to produce the appropriate macronutrient ratios. A common recipe includes stir-frying a variety of vibrant veggies, a lean protein (such as tempeh or chicken), and a portion of whole grains (such as quinoa or brown rice). On the other hand, satisfying and well-rounded meals can be achieved with macro-friendly bowls that include a range of veggies, a protein source, and healthy fats like avocado or olive oil. These choices accommodate a variety of dietary preferences by meeting nutritional needs as well as providing flavor and cooking method flexibility.

DESSERTS AND SNACKS

There is space for indulgence in macrobiotic meal planning as well, but only in moderation. Snacks, which include things like Greek yogurt with berries, a handful of nuts, or an energy bar high in protein, are meant to fill the space between meals. These options help you meet your daily macronutrient targets in addition to satisfying cravings. In the world of macrobiotics, desserts can be tasty and nourishing. For example, a fruit and yogurt parfait or a protein-rich chocolate chia pudding are good options for people who want a treat but still meet their macronutrient goals because they are sweet but not overly so.

Macrorobotic meal planning is a systematic approach to nutrition, with a focus on maintaining a balance of macronutrients in each dish. The emphasis is on developing tasty and filling meals that support individual dietary objectives and enhance general well-being, from breakfast to snacks and sweets.

When creating macrobiotic meals, several elements must be carefully taken into account to guarantee that each person's nutritional needs are satisfied while also taking into account dietary restrictions and addressing specific health issues.

Taking dietary constraints into consideration is important, as these can differ greatly from person to person. It's crucial to modify macrobiotic meal programs to individual preferences or medical concerns.

TAKING CARE OF DIETARY RESTRICTIONS

Dietary limitations can involve avoiding particular foods or substances, and this is especially important to consider while organizing macrobiotic meals. For example, people with celiac disease or gluten intolerance need gluten-free choices. Wheat and other grains include a protein called gluten, which might respond negatively to people who have sensitivity issues. Thankfully, there are lots of gluten-free macrobiotic choices out today, so people with these dietary limitations may still have a varied, nutrient-dense diet.

OPTIONS FOR GLUTEN-FREE MACROBIOTICS

It's crucial to use gluten-free grains in place of regular ones when creating macrobiotic dishes for people with gluten sensitivity. Excellent options that not only supply necessary nutrients but also enhance the overall harmony of a macrobiotic diet include quinoa, brown rice, and buckwheat.

A diverse range of fruits, vegetables, and legumes can be included to ensure a delicious and savory meal while also improving the nutritional profile.

Taking allergens into account is another crucial aspect of macrobiotic meal preparation, in addition to gluten limitations. From widespread allergies to nuts and shellfish to more specialized sensitivity to particular fruits or vegetables, food allergies can take many different forms. The secret is to prepare macrobiotic meals that are high in nutrients and low in allergies. Careful selection and substitution of ingredients may be necessary to preserve the intended macronutrient balance while preserving flavor and nutritional value.

AUTOMATED SYSTEMS FOR ALLERGIES

Paying great attention to ingredient labels and having a solid awareness of potential cross-contamination concerns are generally necessary when using robotic meal planning for allergies. Developing a broad menu that takes into account different types of allergies guarantees that those with particular sensitivity can fully engage in a macrobiotic diet without risking their health.

A key component of macrobiotic meal preparation is inclusivity, which aims to offer options that satisfy a range of dietary requirements. Macrobiotic meals are accessible and delicious for anyone, thanks to careful product selection and meal preparation that takes into account dietary restrictions such as gluten intolerances and particular allergies. The intention is to establish a setting where people with various dietary limitations can nevertheless enjoy the health benefits of macrobiotics, fostering nutritional balance and general well-being.

CHAPTER SIX
MACROSCOPIC WAY OF LIFE
WORKOUT AND MOBILITY

Within the field of Macrobiotic Lifestyle, movement, and exercise are emphasized as essential elements for reaching overall well-being. By adopting an efficient and optimized way of living, people are urged to match their physical activity with the principles of Macrobiotics. To improve overall productivity and vitality, this calls for a strategic approach to exercise that transcends routine and seamlessly incorporates movement into everyday life.

The Macrobiotic Lifestyle views exercise as a continual, harmonious interaction with one's physical body rather than just as a set period set aside for choreographed activities. This method, which emphasizes incorporating movement into everyday activities, is in line with the efficiency ethos. Physical activity is effortlessly incorporated into daily life in Macrobiotic living, as seen by small gestures like stretching during work breaks or choosing to use the stairs rather than the elevator.

CONNECTING EXERCISE TO MACROBOTIC PRINCIPLES

The Macrobiotic Lifestyle emphasizes the importance of selecting an exercise regimen that aligns with personal interests and objectives. Instead of following general, one-size-fits-all methods, people are urged to experiment and learn about a variety of physical activities. Exercises like yoga, strength training, aerobics, and even non-traditional disciplines like dance or martial arts may fall under this category. To ensure long-term adherence and enjoyment, the secret is to choose a regimen that not only advances physical fitness but also fits in with personal interests.

CHOOSING THE PROPER WORKOUT PROGRAM

Furthermore, the Macrobiotic approach to exercise integrates mindfulness, urging participants to be fully present in the moment throughout physical activity. This mindfulness promotes a heightened awareness of one's body and movement throughout the day, extending beyond the gym or set exercise period. By combining mindfulness with physical activity, individuals can get more benefits, not just in terms of physical health but also mental well-being, harmonizing with the overarching concepts of the Macrobiotic Lifestyle.

Exercise and Movement in the Macrobiotic Lifestyle transcend conventional notions of structured workouts, evolving into a seamless integration of physical activity into daily life. The emphasis on aligning with Macrobiotic principles underscores the importance of efficiency, individualization, and mindfulness in crafting the right exercise routine. Through this holistic approach, individuals can not only achieve physical fitness but also cultivate a sustainable and fulfilling lifestyle in tune with the tenets of Macrobiotic living.

MIND-BODY CONNECTION

In the realm of Macrobiotic Lifestyle, the concept of the Mind-Body Connection takes center stage, emphasizing the intricate interplay between mental and physical well-being. Recognizing the profound impact of thoughts and emotions on bodily health, individuals embrace practices that foster harmony between mind and body. This holistic approach underscores the importance of maintaining a balanced and synchronized relationship between cognitive processes and physical states, ultimately contributing to overall well-being.

MEDITATION AND STRESS REDUCTION

Meditation emerges as a cornerstone in the pursuit of a harmonious Mind-Body Connection within the Macrobotic Lifestyle. In this context, meditation transcends its traditional roots, evolving into a futuristic practice that seamlessly integrates technology and mindfulness. Individuals engage in immersive digital experiences that facilitate deep introspection and self-awareness, utilizing advanced biofeedback mechanisms to enhance meditation outcomes. The fusion of ancient contemplative practices with cutting-edge technology represents a unique synthesis that resonates with the ethos of Macrobiotic living.

Stress reduction, a perpetual concern in modern life, finds a bespoke solution in the Macrobiotic Lifestyle through meditation and other innovative practices. The integration of artificial intelligence and biofeedback technologies enables individuals to identify stress triggers and respond proactively. Automated stress-reducing interventions, personalized based on individual preferences and physiological responses, redefine the landscape of emotional well-being. By leveraging the power of Macrobiotics, individuals can cultivate resilience in the face of stressors, fostering a state of mental equilibrium.

EMOTIONAL WELL-BEING IN MACROBIOTICS

Emotional well-being in the context of Macrobiotics transcends the traditional understanding of emotions. It encompasses a nuanced and technologically augmented approach to emotional intelligence. Advanced algorithms and machine learning models analyze emotional patterns, providing insights into individual and collective emotional landscapes. This data-driven understanding facilitates the development of personalized strategies for emotional regulation and enhancement. Macrobiotic Lifestyle envisions a future where emotional well-being is not merely reactive but is actively nurtured through a symbiotic relationship with intelligent technologies.

The Macrobiotic Lifestyle redefines the paradigms of Mind-Body Connection, meditation, and emotional well-being. It envisions a future where individuals seamlessly integrate technology into their pursuit of holistic wellness, leveraging the power of Macrobiotics to enhance self-awareness, reduce stress, and cultivate a profound sense of emotional equilibrium. Through this amalgamation of ancient wisdom and futuristic innovation, Macrobiotic living offers a holistic framework for individuals to thrive in the fast-paced, technologically driven landscapes of the future.